What Every Caregiver or Patient Advocate Should Know

by Kathy Mays Smith

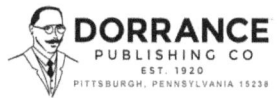

DORRANCE PUBLISHING CO
EST. 1920
PITTSBURGH, PENNSYLVANIA 15238

The contents of this work, including, but not limited to, the accuracy of events, people, and places depicted; opinions expressed; permission to use previously published materials included; and any advice given or actions advocated are solely the responsibility of the author, who assumes all liability for said work and indemnifies the publisher against any claims stemming from publication of the work.

All Rights Reserved
Copyright © 2018 by Kathy Mays Smith

No part of this book may be reproduced or transmitted, downloaded, distributed, reverse engineered, or stored in or introduced into any information storage and retrieval system, in any form or by any means, including photocopying and recording, whether electronic or mechanical, now known or hereinafter invented without permission in writing from the publisher or author.

Dorrance Publishing Co
585 Alpha Drive
Suite 103
Pittsburgh, PA 15238
Visit our website at *www.dorrancebookstore.com*

ISBN: 978-1-4809-8751-7
eISBN: 978-1-4809-8866-8

Introduction

When you take care of a patient, ask yourself, "What would I want if I were that patient? How would I want to be treated?" Remember, the chances are high that that patient was once a vibrant, healthy individual, who had a clear mind, good health, and contributed to society. The following are instructions derived from either the CNA (Certified Nurse Assistant) not doing it right or not doing it. These items are important. Learn them right the first time!

Note:
He = he or she
His = his or hers
Himself = himself or herself

Contents

ADLs 1
ADMINISTRATION OF MEDS 1
AIR CONDITIONER 3
BASICS 5
BED RAILS 5
BRUSHING TEETH AND FLOSSING . . . 7
ENTERING ROOM 9
EYEGLASSES 9
HEARING AIDS 11
INDIVIDUAL INSTRUCTIONS 13
LAUNDRY 13
LIGHTS 15
PATIENT TRANSFER 15
SHOWER 17
SLEEPWEAR 21
TOILETRIES 21
TOWELS 21
URINAL 23
A LITTLE TLC 29
VISITORS 33
DOCUMENT 37

ADLs (Activities for Daily Living): Patients will vary in their need for help in dressing. Do not pull socks tightly over toes. After putting them on, loosen socks slightly at the toes. The patient may or may not be able to button shirt or put on shoes. Assist where necessary.

ADMINISTRATION OF MEDS: If the patient is given medications in bed, be sure that the head of the bed is sufficiently elevated. Some patients must have thickened water or take medications with applesauce. Be sure to find out what applies to your patient. Make sure the patient has swallowed all his medications before you leave the room. Otherwise, especially if he has a swallowing problem, he may choke or develop aspiration pneumonia, which can be fatal.

Notes

AIR CONDITIONER: Some of the air conditioners at the facility may very old. If the room is too hot or too cold, report it to the nurse. It may not be functioning. Or someone other than the patient may have turned it off. Some units may require a towel to control the amount of hot or cold air that comes out. Find what the patient wants. The room should be a comfortable temperature. Make sure if the patient wants the door open, partially open, or closed. If wide open and the hall is hot, it will make the room too hot. If closed, it may make the room too cold. This will vary from room to room.

Notes

BASICS: Answer the **call button** ASAP. If you are chatting with another staff member, respond to that patient now, not later. You've answered a call button. You are with the patient. Your gizmo that buzzes you tells you two other patients have hit their call buttons. What do you do? No matter what, be sure that the patient you are with can reach his **call button, the bed remote, the light cord/switch, and phone** before you leave the room. If necessary, go back and make sure that there is drinking water available and that the bedside tray is within reach. For some patients, water may have to be thickened. Whatever you do, do not turn off the call button until you have finished helping the patient.

BED RAILS: When the patient is in bed, the bed rails should always be elevated.

Notes

BRUSHING TEETH AND FLOSSING: See whether the patient can brush his own teeth. If there is an electric toothbrush, have him use it rather than a plain toothbrush to keep gums healthy. Afterward, floss teeth. If the patient cannot do it himself, assist him. If not provided, there is an electric "airflosser," which can shoot air in spurts at the gum line between the teeth toward the tongue and gets residual debris that an ordinary flossing does not. The patient or family can check with the dentist or pharmacist about this. When brushing teeth, cover the patient with a towel from neck down and across his lap. This saves from soiling clothing with toothpaste and saliva. Put the electric toothbrush on its charger. Be sure you place it correctly. If jammed on backward, it could damage the toothbrush and charger.

Notes

ENTERING ROOM: Before entering the room, knock on the door quietly, so if the patient is asleep, he won't be wakened. Constant interruptions can leave a patient exhausted. If they have a certain period posted "Do not disturb," you are not an exception. It means you, too. Respect that.

EYEGLASSES: If family doesn't clean glasses, clean them so they will be clean the next morning (or sooner, if splattered). Do not wipe with Kleenex or a paper towel. There should be special lens cleaner and a soft cloth. Paper will scratch the lens. Learn what the family wants in this respect.

Notes

HEARING AIDS: There are many kinds of hearing aids, but it is universal to have a red marking on the one for the right ear. Make sure they are removed before shower or before patient goes to bed. Make sure ears are dry before putting them back in the patient's ears. If the patient has a special receptacle to place them, be sure they are put there. Make sure the hearing aid is securely in place and the "wire" fits inside the curve of the ear. When taking them off, check to see if the battery is good: Rubbing the part that fits behind the ear and hearing a paper rustling sound means the battery is good. No noise means the battery is dead and should be replaced. Make sure the hearing aid is open while not worn by the patient. Before replacing in the ear, make sure you have put the battery in with the flat side up. Make sure the hearing aid "clicks" when closed.

Notes

INDIVIDUAL INSTRUCTIONS: The family may have special instructions. Be sure to read them until the information becomes automatic. Notes may be pinned on clothing for the next day or may be on the sign-in tray, where you have signed the time you have assisted the patient and what you did.

LAUNDRY: There are bags furnished by the facility for laundry, if done there. If done by the family, put wet clothing in a plastic bag before putting it in a laundry basket or container that the family has for laundry. If you don't know, ask the unit manager or nurse.

Notes

LIGHTS: Lights may be turned on with a pull cord or a switch. Be sure the patient can reach it and knows where it is. If it's behind his head and out of reach, you can tie the cord to the rail of the bed where the patient can reach it. If a door is closed and no light has been left on, such a situation can become very frightening to the patient when he needs help.

PATIENT TRANSFER: In transferring a patient from bed to wheelchair, to toilet, from toilet, etc., have him use the handrails of the bed. Guide him with sitting and standing. Some patients may try to sit down before they get to the proper position. Help the patient sit up and dress, if necessary. This will vary with different patients.

Notes

SHOWER: Have clothes, shampoo, deodorant, and clean clothing with you when you take the patient to the shower. Do not leave him to go get them. Sheets should be changed before or after the shower, but do not allow the patient to sit uncovered and wet in front of the air conditioner or cool room.

Learn how the patient likes pillows: stacked, layered, at shoulders or above, etc. The same with bedding: Avoid folding back the blanket in an extra layer around the neck or chest. This can cause sweating. Make sure you have two sheets on the bed, a facility or personal blanket, transfer sheet, and pillows in place. The patient may want or have an additional blanket.

Notes

(Shower, cont.)

Always dry between toes after shower. If using body powder, be sure the skin is dry enough that the powder doesn't cake and stick to body and clothing.

Body soap provided by facility, if used as shampoo, may cause dandruff. Check to see if there are special instructions and shampoos. Apply patient's deodorant. Brush or comb patient's hair while it is still wet. Find out how the patient likes to have his hair brushed. Grooming is important, and the hair will dry looking nice and not rumpled the next day.

Notes

SLEEPWEAR: The patient may prefer pajamas or just a T-shirt and may or may not want to sleep in sleepwear pants. Ask. If yes, make sure pant legs are pulled down to ankles and (for men) fly is in front. Make sure shirt is smooth on the back. It gets uncomfortable to sleep on wrinkles.

TOILETRIES: Learn where the patient keeps toiletries and see that they are placed back in an orderly fashion after use.

TOWELS: Be sure that towels and washcloths are in the room. Each patient may want them placed a different way. Some patients like to keep a towel on the seat of wheelchair to protect it from food, soiling, etc.

Notes

URINAL: The patient may be unable to make it to the bathroom by himself and need assistance. If the request is for a urinal, the urinal should be close to the bed, in reaching distance if the patient is able to perform the function by himself. If not, be sure that the urinal does not lie there, tilted, and back end up—this will result in pouring urine on the patient and diaper or other clothing when the urinal is removed. Give the patient time. Sometimes it takes a minute or two for the flow to begin.

Have dry diaper/pull-up at hand. Do not walk out to get something without covering the patient and allowing him a degree of privacy. Do not leave the door wide open for all passersby to see him unclothed. Never take diapers from one room to another patient. It may be that family is providing and paying for them.

Notes

(Urinal, cont.)

If the patient was wet, clean with perianal wipes. Always make sure that a good supply of wipes is close at hand. Use these wipes to clean the incontinent person in incontinent care. Stock room with wipes so they are available for aide to use. Protect privacy—close the door or pull the privacy curtain if providing peri care. If the storeroom is out or low, contact the nurse. Never let the patient become "stinky." Take the urinal into the bathroom. Raise the toilet seat. Pour the contents into the toilet. Pull down the spray attachment and rinse the urinal thoroughly. Rinse again. Empty. Empty remaining drops a few seconds later. Put spray attachment back up and toilet seat down. Do not place lid on urinal. Return it to original spot and leave to air dry.

Notes

(Urinal, cont.)

Dementia patients may need encouragement. Just offering a urinal every two hours may not be enough. Explain that it's been two hours, that using it now prevents wetting the diaper and reduces chance of infection or that the family wants him to do it. Parkinson's patients decline over time. What they could do before, suddenly or not so suddenly, they may not be able to do now.

If a diaper has been wet, check clothing and sheets to be sure that they have not been wet also. If so, change clothing and sheets. Never tuck a shirt into a pull-up or diaper. If the pull-up or diaper gets wet, a tucked-in shirt will get wet also.

Notes

A LITTLE TLC: Family members will appreciate being updated on the patient's day: Did he have his shower? If tending to become constipated, did he have a bowel movement? Does he seem better? Worse? Needs? If you are going on your break, let the family know and when you expect to be back.

If the mattress has slipped down, get help and pull the mattress back up to the headboard. If the patient has slipped down, have another aide help you use the transfer sheet to pull him back up. In elevating the bed or lowering it, do moves in increments and ask the patient to tell you when "it's good." Do not leave patient with feet off the side of bed.

If you are in the room and the phone rings, answer it for the patient. Make sure he is holding it properly and can hear the other

Notes

(A Little TLC, cont.)

person before you leave the room, especially in dementia cases. In those cases, go back to make sure the phone has been placed back on the phone "hook."

If you notice a wound bleeding, perhaps puffiness of lips, red eyelid, or something unusual about the patient, report it to the nurse. It may be an allergic reaction or adverse side-effect to a new medication.

When bringing the patient back from the dining room or elsewhere, offer the urinal or trip to the toilet. Then offer to turn on the TV and ask what he would like to watch. Be sure the volume isn't so high that it damages his hearing. Leave the TV remote within his reach on the bedside tray.

Always make sure there is water in a container the patient can reach and drink.

Notes

VISITORS: But as important or even more so, visitors and activities the patient can still do can fill the patient's days with purpose and fulfillment. Days blur into each other, and keeping apprised of current events helps. Laughter is the best medicine, and sharing a joke is rewarding.

A hospital or nursing facility can be a very lonely place. Friends become uncertain how to act or perceive a deteriorating mental condition and become uncomfortable and stop coming. The visitor doesn't have to have an agenda—tell about a current event or just listen to the patient. Ask the patient about experiences that can be written up and shared with the family. Tell about his life, perhaps his military service, his dreams, ambitions, or miracles he may have experienced that he may appreciate being recorded for family.

Notes

(Visitors, cont.)

If the patient can no longer read, there are free audio books available from the State. Reading some each day gives the patient something to look forward to. Fact or fiction—or a mixture of both! Perhaps he would enjoy a Bible study.

If the patient is in pain, he may prefer no visitors. There may be only certain hours visitors are allowed. They should be honored.

If the patient is strong enough, see if he can be taken out to dinner or a movie or some beautiful park. Nothing becomes more of a prison than being cooped up in the same room without break day after day.

In spite of the negatives, the final days or years can be rewarding for the patient and his family and friends. The caregiver or advocate can be and is an instrument to achieve this.

Notes

DOCUMENT: It is a good idea to document—the name of the nurse(s) and CNAs on duty, i.e. who gives the medications that day. Research potential new drugs to see if there is a conflict with medicines the patient is taking or if he has a history of negative effects from a medicine that is contraindicated before giving permission to give it to the patient. The doctor may be rushed and not do the research of records to see what allergies the patient may have.

It is unfortunate, but a reality, that something actually malpractice may be placed in the category of "incident report" for training of employees. In such case, it may never show on the medical records, and in the worst-case scenario legal recourse is useless. In asking for medical records, it won't be in them. If you suspect malpractice, report it immediately to an attorney.

Notes

www.ingramcontent.com/pod-product-compliance
Lightning Source LLC
Chambersburg PA
CBHW061520180526
45171CB00001B/268